explaining...
DIABETES

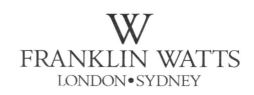

W

FRANKLIN WATTS
LONDON • SYDNEY

ANITA LOUGHREY

First published in 2008 by
Franklin Watts
338 Euston Road
London NW1 3BH

Franklin Watts Australia
Level 17/207 Kent Street
Sydney NSW 2000

© 2008 Franklin Watts

ISBN 978 07496 8259 0

Dewey classification number: 618.92'462

Planning and production by Discovery Books Limited
Managing Editor: Laura Durman
Editor: Annabel Savery
Designer: Keith Williams
Picture research: Rachel Tisdale
Consultant: Kathryn McCrea, Consultant Paediatrician with an interest in Diabetes, Shrewsbury and Telford Hospitals NHS Trust

Printed in China

Franklin Watts is a division of Hachette Children's Books, an Hachette Livre Company.
www.hachettelivre.co.uk

Photo acknowledgements: Barbara Durman: p. 39; Corbis: p. 31 (Thom Lang); Discovery Picture Library: front cover bottom left (Chris Fairclough), 22 (Chris Fairclough), 27, (Chris Fairclough), 28 (Chris Fairclough); Getty Images: p. 29 (Jamie McDonald); istockphoto.com: pp. 20, 23 (Michal Kram), 30 right (Sergey Lavrentev), 36 (Aldo Murillo); John Birdsall Photo Library/www.JohnBirdsall.co.uk: front cover top, front cover bottom right, pp. 8, 12, 16, 32, 34, 37; www.levity.com: p. 10; Science Photo Library: pp. 18 (Lea Paterson), 19 (Custom Medical Stock Photo), 21 (Cordelia Molloy), 30 left (Adam Gault); Science and Society Picture Library: p. 11; Shutterstock: pp. 14 (Lisa F Young), 17 (Anetta), 26, 33 (Photobank)

Source credits: We would like to thank the following for their contribution: www.dyslexia-teacher.co.uk; www.steveredgrave.com; Cathy Gowland.

Please note the case studies in this book are either true life stories or based on true life stories.

The pictures in the book feature a mixture of adults and children with and without diabetes. Some of the photographs feature models, and it should not be implied that they have diabetes.

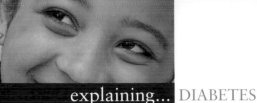

Contents

What is diabetes?

Diabetes is a condition where people are unable to control the level of glucose – a type of sugar – in their blood because their pancreas does not work properly. It is not contagious and is invisible. People with diabetes look like everybody else.

How many people have diabetes?

There are 246 million people worldwide who have been diagnosed with diabetes and it has been estimated that it will affect 380 million by 2025. Worldwide, as many as 440,000 children and adolescents under the age of 15 have diabetes. At least 50 per cent of all people with diabetes are unaware of their condition. If people have not been diagnosed then they will not be receiving the necessary treatment. In some countries this figure may reach 80 per cent.

Types of diabetes

There are two main types of diabetes, Type 1 and Type 2 diabetes. They affect different people and have different causes. In both cases, the body is unable to control the level of glucose in the blood. Type 1 and 2 diabetes are explained in more detail on pages 12-15.

How the pancreas works

The pancreas is a small gland about 15 cm long, which lies crosswise behind the stomach. Under normal circumstances, the pancreas produces a hormone called insulin that controls the amount of glucose in the blood. Insulin is produced by groups of cells inside the pancreas known as the islets of Langerhans.

▼ *Any of the children in this picture could have diabetes. You cannot tell if someone has diabetes just by looking at them.*

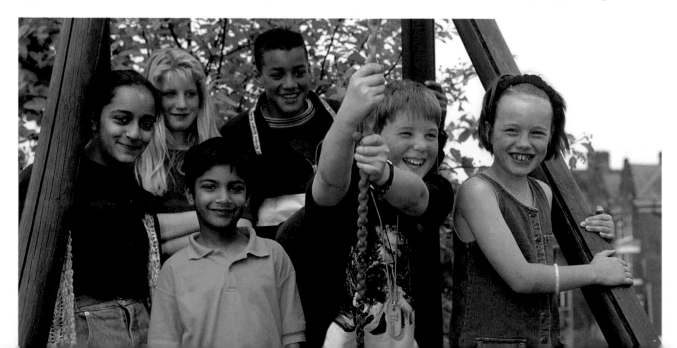

► *The beta cells in the islets of Langerhans in the pancreas produce insulin.*

Insulin converts glucose from food into energy to be used by the body. Glucose is found in carbohydrates, such as bread products, cereals, rice, potatoes, yams and plantain, as well as in sugar and other sweet foods. Insulin also helps the liver absorb and store glucose that is not being used immediately. When the body needs energy, the liver releases glucose into the bloodstream and insulin then helps the body to turn the glucose into energy. This keeps blood glucose levels stable. One of the first signs of diabetes may be frequent urination (see page 17).

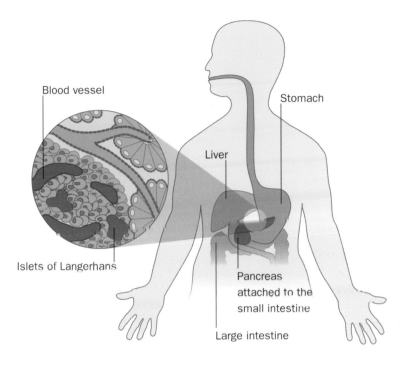

Blood vessel

Stomach

Liver

Islets of Langerhans

Pancreas attached to the small intestine

Large intestine

People with diabetes

When someone has diabetes, the body produces either too little insulin or none at all. Without enough insulin, the body is unable to turn glucose from food into energy. This means blood glucose levels may become too high or too low, and help is needed to maintain healthy glucose levels.

Who has diabetes?

Diabetes may result from a combination of hereditary and environmental factors, such as what and how much a person eats and how much exercise they do. Studies of identical twins have shown that if one twin develops diabetes, the other twin is likely to as well.

Research has shown that diabetes is more common in women than men. There are also marked differences in the development of diabetes between ethnic groups. People from the Asian

community are six times more likely to develop Type 2 diabetes than Caucasian people; and those whose origins are African-Caribbean are three times more likely.

PEOPLE AT RISK OF DIABETES

Some people are more at risk of developing diabetes than others. These are some of the factors that might affect a person's likelihood of developing diabetes.

• Family history • Age • Ethnicity • Weight
• Waist measurement • Blood pressure
• Previous medical conditions.

Some people may have only one of these factors, others may have many.

Diabetes: a brief history

The first known mention of diabetes was in 1500 BCE when an Egyptian doctor called Hesy-Ra gave advice on the treatment of frequent urination in the Ebers Papyrus. The next record of diabetes is found 1600 years later in 100 CE when Aretaeus of Cappadocia, a Greek doctor, named the condition of frequent urination diabetes, meaning 'flowing through'. He described diabetes as 'the melting down of flesh and limbs into urine'.

Taste test

In the 16th century, a Swiss doctor called Paracelsus noticed a white powder that he thought was salt in the evaporated urine of a diabetic patient. This white powder was actually sugar. It was not until 100 years later that someone tasted a urine sample and noticed it was sweet. After this the condition became known as diabetes mellitus, as 'mellitus' means 'sweet as honey'.

Islets of Langerhans

In 1869 Paul Langerhans, a German medical student, found the groups of islet cells in the pancreas that are named after him. They are known as the 'islets of Langerhans' because they look like little islands under the microscope.

In 1910 Sir Edward Sharpey-Schafer, an English physiologist, suggested that the pancreas in people

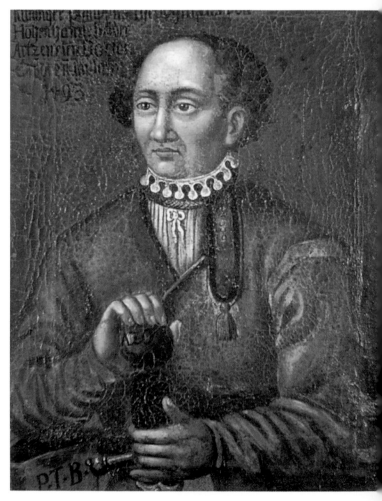

▶ *Paracelsus was born in 1493 in Einsiedeln, Switzerland. He was the first to identify diabetes as a serious disorder.*

with diabetes did not produce a chemical as it normally would. In 1916 the beta cells in the islets of Langerhans were identified as the source of a hormone. A few years later, in 1921, Canadians Dr Frederick Banting and his assistant, Charles Best, gave this hormone to an eleven-year-old named Leonard Thompson in an injection. They found that regular injections lowered his blood glucose level. This hormone was named insulin.

Taking insulin

Once the importance of insulin was discovered, scientists had to find ways for people to take it. In 1944, the standard syringe was introduced to help diabetics inject insulin. The advances in DNA technology between 1950 and 1980 meant that genetically engineered 'human' insulin was made available, and since then other forms of insulin have been introduced. In 1959 the two types of diabetes were recognised: Type 1 (insulin-dependent) diabetes and Type 2 (non-insulin-dependent) diabetes. Tablets were also introduced to help lower blood glucose levels for those with Type 2 diabetes.

Testing blood glucose levels

In the 1960s, home testing for glucose levels in urine gave diabetics an increased level of control over their condition, and since the 1980s people have been able to test their blood glucose level at home using blood glucose meters. Now there are different types of blood glucose meters and the doctor can help to decide which is best for each patient. Technological innovations have also made controlling diabetes much easier. The insulin auto-pen delivery system was introduced in 1986, which meant children and young people were able to take their insulin easily at school.

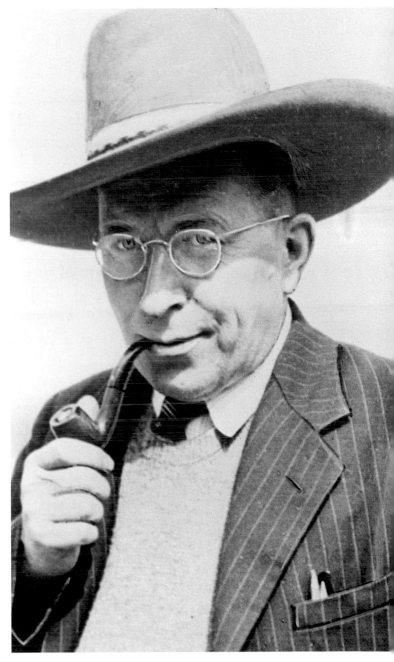

▲ *Dr Frederick Banting was the first person to experiment with injecting insulin. After Dr Banting discovered insulin, it was put into mass production within months and immediately began to extend the lives of millions of people with diabetes.*

Type 1 diabetes

Type 1 diabetes is sometimes called 'insulin dependent diabetes mellitus' (IDDM) because the body is unable to produce its own insulin and so is dependent on insulin injections.

Causes of Type 1 diabetes

Type 1 diabetes occurs when the body has destroyed the cells in the pancreas that produce insulin. Scientists do not know exactly why the body destroys these cells, it may be that the body has had an abnormal reaction to them because of a viral or other infection.

Type 1 diabetes is most commonly diagnosed during childhood or teenage years, but can occur later in life, normally before the age of 40. Type 1 diabetes is less common than Type 2 and accounts for between 5-15 per cent of all people with diabetes. However, the number of young people in the world with Type 1 diabetes is steadily increasing.

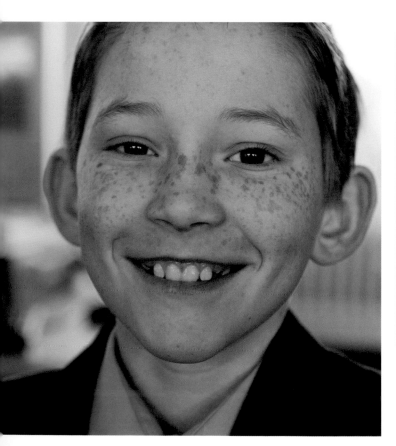

RATES OF INCREASE

Type 1 diabetes is growing by three per cent per year in children and adolescents, and at an alarming five per cent per year among pre-school children. It is estimated that 70,000 children under the age of 15 develop Type 1 diabetes each year (almost 200 children a day). Of the estimated 440,000 cases of Type 1 diabetes in children worldwide, more than a quarter live in South-east Asia and more than a fifth in Europe.

◀ *Type 1 diabetes is usually diagnosed during childhood or teenage years. In Type 1 diabetes the body relies on injections of insulin.*

LEE'S STORY

Lee is 13 years old and has Type 1 diabetes. He was diagnosed when he was 18 months old. 'My mum says I was extremely thirsty, drinking loads and wetting loads of nappies. She knew something was wrong.

'My parents told the doctor my symptoms and the first thing he did was a urine test, which showed I had too much sugar in my urine. Then they had to do blood tests. I was very young so I don't remember very much about it. The blood tests showed I definitely had diabetes. I have grown up having injections and they are just a part of my everyday life. At first my parents used to do them for me. I started to do my own injections when I was about nine years old.'

Lee monitors his blood glucose levels three or four times a day, usually first thing in the morning, after lunch, after school and last thing at night. 'To monitor my own glucose levels I use a blood glucose meter. First I put a blood glucose strip into the meter. Then I prick my finger using a special device that does not let the needle go in too deep. I squeeze a drop of blood onto the strip and the machine shows me what my blood glucose levels are. If I feel like my blood glucose is low I test more often and drink full sugar drinks.'

Lee sees a consultant four times a year. The consultant does a blood test that gives a measure of his average blood glucose level during the last 2-3 months. This gives an indication of how well he is controlling his glucose levels.

Lee also has an annual check-up with a specialist nurse who does a blood test, checks his blood pressure and looks at his injection sites. He also has a chat with a dietician and has retinal screening annually too, because diabetes can cause problems with the eyes (see pages 22 and 23). To control his diabetes he takes four injections every day, using two different types of insulin.

Having diabetes does not stop Lee joining in at school and he enjoys playing sport. 'I do PE twice a week and football training and matches weekly. I eat glucose tablets before PE and have extra food after football.'

In Type 1 diabetes, the body does not produce insulin, so the glucose in the blood cannot be converted into energy. Instead it builds up, causing high blood glucose levels. If left untreated high blood glucose can cause serious long-term health problems (see pages 22-25). The normal treatment for people with Type 1 diabetes is daily injections of insulin which keep the blood sugar levels within normal ranges. There are different types of insulin and each person will have to work out which type works best for them.

Type 2 diabetes

Type 2 diabetes is described as 'non-insulin-dependent diabetes mellitus' (NIDDM). It is the most common form of diabetes, accounting for between 85-95 per cent of all people with diabetes.

What causes Type 2 diabetes?

This type of diabetes usually appears later in life, often between the age of 35-45 years, and is sometimes called mature-onset diabetes. However, recently, increasing numbers of children are being diagnosed with the condition, some as young as seven.

In Type 2 diabetes, the body either produces too little insulin, which means it cannot convert enough glucose into energy, or it is insulin resistant, which means it does not use insulin correctly. If a body cannot use insulin correctly then the amount of insulin produced will have less of an effect, and less glucose will be converted into energy. The body needs to produce more and more insulin to be able to convert the same amount of glucose into energy. In both cases, as the body is unable to convert glucose into energy, it builds up in the bloodstream instead of going into the cells.

▼ *Type 2 diabetes used to be a condition that only affected older people, but it now affects many young children too.*

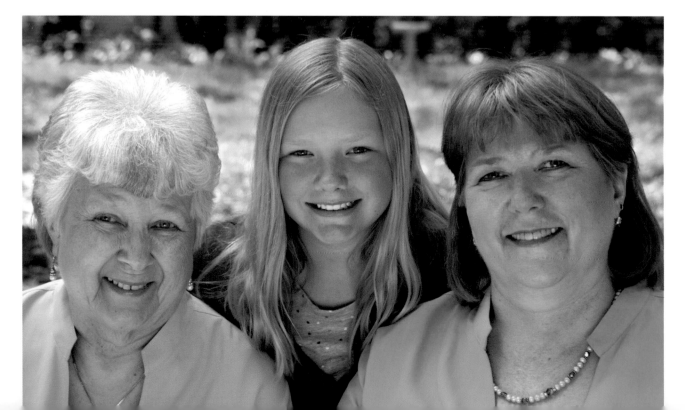

Being overweight

In most cases Type 2 diabetes is linked with being overweight. Many researchers believe that the increase in cases of Type 2 diabetes in children is linked to the rise in childhood obesity. Overweight people have lots of fat cells in their bodies which are more resistant to insulin than muscle cells. The pancreas usually responds to this by producing more insulin. This can go on for a long time, sometimes many years. Eventually the pancreas is unable to continue producing the high amounts of insulin needed to keep blood sugar levels normal. Up to 80 per cent of cases of Type 2 diabetes are preventable by adopting a healthy diet and increasing physical activity.

As Type 2 diabetes develops slowly, many people do not recognise the symptoms and do not realise they have diabetes. If left untreated, high blood glucose can cause serious long-term health problems (see pages 22-25).

INCREASE IN TYPE 2 DIABETES

Around the world, Type 2 diabetes is increasing in young people. In some areas of the USA as many as 45 per cent of children newly diagnosed with diabetes have Type 2. Over a 20-year period, instances of Type 2 diabetes have doubled in children in Japan. Diabetes has also risen in young Native Americans and Australian Aborigines, which may reflect a change in their diet and lifestyle.

CASE NOTES

SAMANTHA'S STORY

Samantha is twelve years old and was diagnosed with Type 2 diabetes last year. 'We discovered I had diabetes because I was always feeling tired and constantly thirsty so my dad took me to the doctor. Now I take tablets every day.'

She does blood sugar checks twice a day using a blood glucose meter and has regular check-ups for her eyes, feet and blood pressure, plus three-monthly blood samples taken at the local hospital. She has to be far more aware of picking up viruses, colds etc because they will affect her glucose levels. 'When I am ill I need to see the doctor as I may need to take different tablets to ensure my glucose levels don't get too high.'

'When I was first diagnosed I felt confused and very resentful. I thought, "Why me?" I did not know what would happen next and thought it would stop me from going out with my friends and having fun. I was especially upset and angry about having to change my diet, but now I have noticed the benefits and understand why it is important.'

Samantha sees a dietician who explains what food she is allowed to eat, 'Mostly the healthy options that are low in fat and low Glycaemic Index (GI) type foods. It is just sensible, healthy eating. This doesn't mean I can't have treats every now and again. The dietician recommends I eat regularly and have something with me, such as a high sugar drink or sweet snacks in case my blood sugar falls too low.'

Symptoms and diagnosis

Most children are diagnosed with diabetes around the ages of ten to thirteen, but not everyone has the same symptoms. Symptoms of Type 1 diabetes are usually very obvious and develop quickly. Symptoms of Type 2 diabetes are not as easy to spot, they can appear slowly and sometimes do not show for a long time. Once a person starts having treatment for diabetes, the symptoms can disappear quickly.

Methods of diagnosis:

If people think they have the symptoms of diabetes they can go to their doctor and ask for a diabetes test. A doctor will do several different tests to make sure the diagnosis is correct.

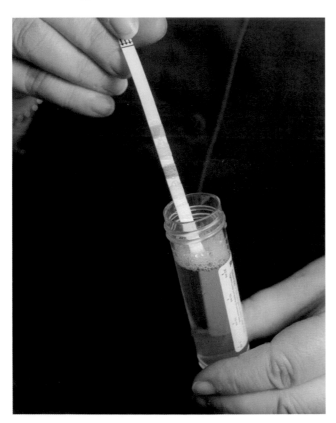

1. Urine test When someone is diabetic the glucose from their food cannot be processed properly, so some will be passed out of the body in urine. High glucose levels in urine are a good indication that someone is diabetic. A sample of urine is tested with a paper dipstick which changes colour according to how much glucose is present. The dipstick is compared to a colour chart to check the result. If the urine contains glucose, further tests are required to confirm the diagnosis.

2. Fingerprick test A special device is used to prick the side of the fingertip and a drop of blood is squeezed onto a testing strip. The strip is put into a blood glucose meter to be analysed. The level of glucose in blood is measured in millimoles per litre. A millimole is a very small measure. A healthy blood glucose level is 4-6 millimoles per litre. If the result is above this, further tests, such as a blood glucose test, are required.

◄ *A paper dipstick is used to test a sample of urine. The dipstick will show the level of sugar in the blood.*

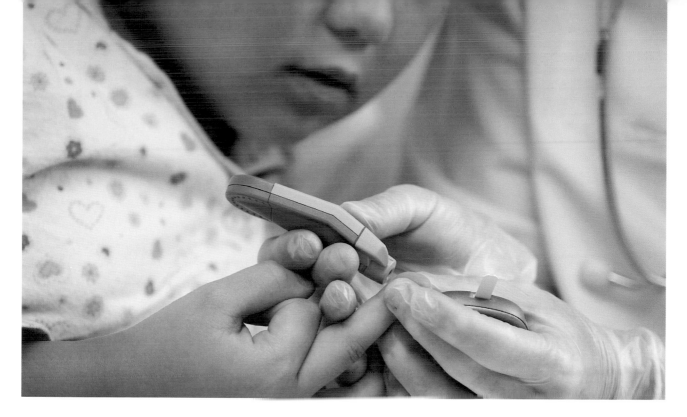

▲ *A fingerprick test is performed on a child to measure the level of glucose in her blood.*

SYMPTOMS

Some of the symptoms of both types of diabetes include:

• Always being thirsty

• Passing large amounts of urine

• Urinary tract infections, such as cystitis

• Fungal infections, such as thrush

• Weight loss

• A lack of energy

• Blurred vision caused by dehydration of the lenses in the eyes

• Fruity-smelling breath

• Dry skin.

3. Blood glucose test A blood sample is taken and sent to a laboratory to test the glucose levels. Results are usually received within a week. If the blood glucose level is above 11.1 millimoles per litre, the patient is diagnosed with diabetes. If it is below this, but the symptoms are still present, a fasting blood glucose test is needed.

4. Fasting blood glucose test The patient does not eat or drink overnight and in the morning a blood test is done. If the test result shows glucose levels are above 7 millimoles per litre, diabetes is confirmed.

5. Oral glucose tolerance test This test is only usually used when other tests have been inconclusive, or when diagnosing diabetes during pregnancy. The patient does not eat or drink overnight and in the morning a blood test is taken before drinking some glucose, and again two hours after drinking the glucose. The blood tests are sent to the laboratory and results are usually received back within a week. If the test result shows glucose levels are above 7 millimoles per litre and the two hour test is above 11.1 millimoles per litre, the patient is diagnosed with diabetes.

Medication

Type 1 diabetes is controlled by insulin. The most effective way of getting insulin into the bloodstream is to inject it. Type 2 diabetes can usually be controlled by a healthy diet, exercise and taking tablets. However, Type 2 diabetics may need to be prescribed insulin if their blood glucose reaches the point where it can no longer be controlled by tablets.

Types of insulin

Insulin types can be split into three groups, human, analogue and animal. Human and analogue insulins are produced synthetically, which means they are produced in a lab. Human insulin is identical to that produced in the body and analogue insulin is almost identical to insulin produced in the body. Animal insulin comes from the pancreas of pigs and cows and works in a very similar way to human insulin.

Different types of insulin work in different ways. The main difference between each type is the amount of time it takes to work in the body after it has been injected. Some types act quickly and wear off after a few hours. Others take longer to start working and last longer, up to ten or 12 hours, some also last up to 24 hours. Diabetics may find one type of insulin suits them, or they may need to use a combination of different ones. Most types of insulin reach a time of peak action when there will be lots of insulin in the blood.

▶ *Nowadays it is quick and easy for a diabetic to inject their own insulin, and there are many different devices that can be used.*

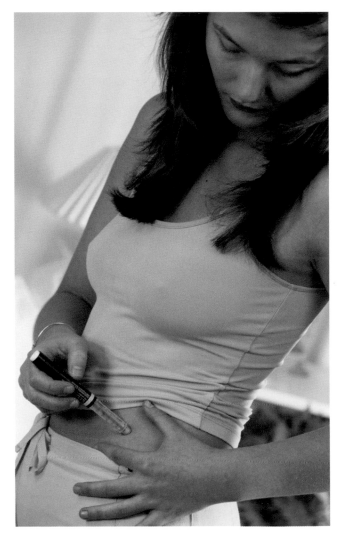

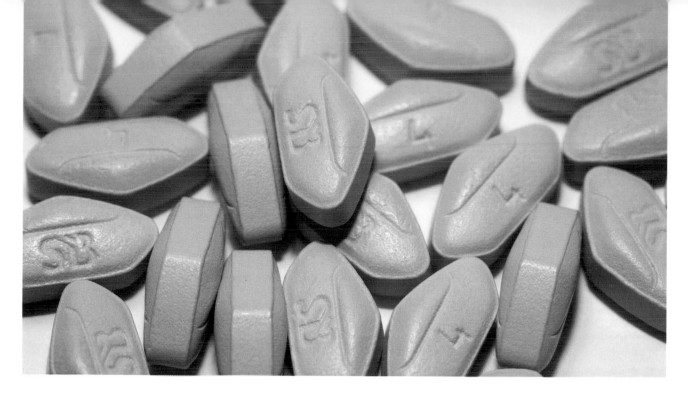

▲ *There is a wide range of tablets that can be prescribed to help people with Type 2 diabetes. The tablets shown here help to increase the body's sensitivity to insulin.*

Diabetics will need to eat something around the time of peak action so that there is enough glucose in the body for the insulin to work on, to prevent glucose levels falling too low.

Regimes

People with diabetes use a regime to organise when they take their insulin. This will depend on the type of insulin that suits them and their lifestyle best.

One of the most common is the basal bolus regime, which uses a combination of long- and short-acting insulin to control blood glucose levels throughout the day. Basal insulin is long-acting and provides a steady supply of insulin for the body to use all day and night. Bolus insulin is short-acting and needs to be taken before meals and big snacks to boost the level of insulin in the blood and help the body to cope with food intake. People on this regime may need to check their blood glucose in the middle of the night once a fortnight to make sure that their blood glucose level does not fall too low during the night.

Where on the body to inject

The thighs, stomach and bottom are the main sites to inject insulin. It is injected under the skin rather than into a vein or muscle. Diabetics should vary the exact position and stay as relaxed as possible. If necessary, diabetics can numb the area with ice for a few minutes. The needles used are very thin and do not usually mark the skin, although sometimes there may be a little bruising or bleeding.

Tablets

Tablets are only prescribed to people with Type 2 diabetes. They are usually taken before or after meals. The tablets are not a form of insulin and do not work in the same way. Insulin cannot be taken orally as it would be destroyed by the stomach before it could work. Diabetes tablets work in different ways to help lower the level of glucose in the blood. Some stimulate the pancreas to produce more insulin, while others help the body to use the insulin it produces more effectively and reduce insulin resistance.

Hypoglycaemia

Hypoglycaemia means 'low blood glucose' and is often abbreviated to 'hypo'.

Hypos occur when there is not enough glucose in the blood. People with diabetes must monitor their bodies to prevent themselves from having hypos.

Effects of hypoglycaemia

If low blood glucose is not treated promptly, it can cause confusion, headaches and irritability. In severe cases a person may lose consciousness. Hypoglycaemia can cause a loss of control over the body and is a distressing experience. Young people will find their mental agility (ability to make decisions) and attention span become limited.

The level at which a person may begin to experience symptoms of hypoglycaemia will change, depending on how often their blood glucose levels have been low over the last few days. As a precaution, diabetics should carry quickly-absorbed glucose snacks or a sweet drink.

SYMPTOMS OF HYPOGLYCAEMIA

Diabetics have to learn to recognise the symptoms of hypoglycaemia. There are two types of symptoms to be aware of, symptoms from the brain and symptoms from the body.

Symptoms of hypoglycaemia from the brain:
- blurred vision
- difficulty concentrating
- poor judgement
- hearing problems
- lack of concentration
- poor memory
- poor co-ordination
- colour blindness
- dizziness
- headache
- anxiety
- seizure

Symptoms of hypoglycaemia from the body:
- hot flushes
- hunger
- paleness
- numb fingers and tongue
- throbbing pulse in chest and stomach
- cold sweats
- nausea
- tingly lips
- trembling

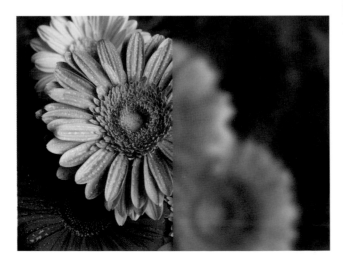

◄ *Half of this picture shows normal vision and the other half shows what it would look like if your vision was blurred. Blurred vision is one of the symptoms of hypoglycaemia.*

Dr Ragnar Hanas in his book, *Type 1 Diabetes in Children, Adolescents and Young Adults* says: 'You should check your blood glucose level whenever you have symptoms or feel strange. This is particularly important in the early days following diagnosis, when you are learning how to recognise your own individual reactions to hypoglycaemia.'

Glucagon

Glucagon is another hormone produced by the pancreas. It raises blood glucose levels by triggering the release of glucose into the bloodstream. Glucagon is only used in an emergency if a diabetic falls unconscious. Glucagon kits are available for home use, usually by prescription. Glucagon kits are a good safety net for parents with a diabetic child.

HAVING A HYPO

This is what one person with diabetes said about having a hypo.

'If I have a hypo, which is very rare nowadays, I feel very hot and sweaty. My hands start to shake and my vision becomes blurry. I've been told I speak too fast and don't make sense. It can happen so quickly and I feel completely disorientated and unable to concentrate on what I am talking about.'

▼ *In an emergency, glucagon can be used to raise blood glucose levels. Glucagon can be given as an injection or with an auto-pen delivery system.*

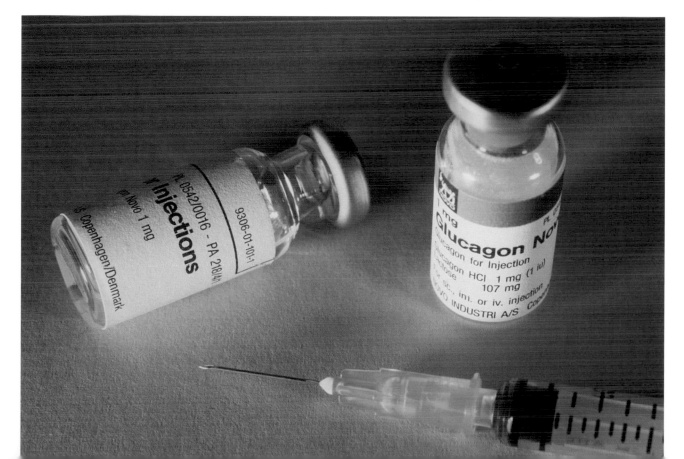

Eyes, skin and feet

People with diabetes are more likely than other people to experience problems with their eyes, skin and feet. They should have good hygiene routines and regular check-ups so that these problems can be avoided.

Eyes

People with diabetes must go for regular eye tests because diabetes can affect the eyes in various ways. It can cause blurred vision, cataracts and diabetic retinopathy. Early detection and treatment can prevent progression of these problems, which in severe cases can lead to blindness.

▼ *It is important that people with diabetes go for regular eye tests, like this one, to prevent serious problems occurring.*

Blurred vision is caused by the lenses in the eyes becoming dehydrated before diabetes is diagnosed. After diagnosis, the onset of treatment may cause a fluid shift in the eyes. This is temporary and should correct itself within a few months. People with diabetes should wait until their condition is stable before going for an eye test to see if they need to be prescribed glasses or contact lenses.

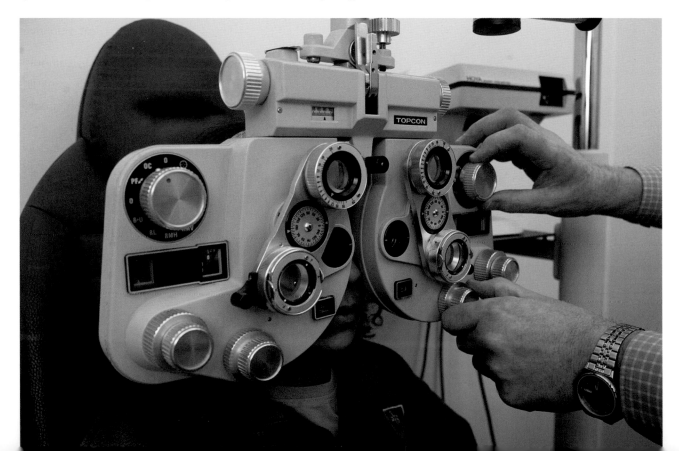

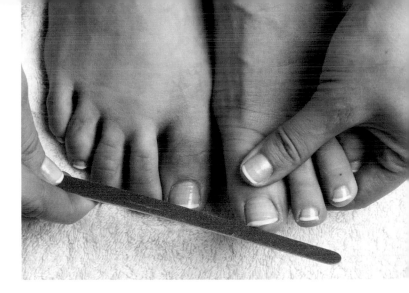

People with diabetes are more susceptible to cataracts because of the build-up of sugars in the lens of the eye. These sugars make the lens of the eye cloudy, interfering with the transmission of light to the back of the eye. A diabetic is particularly sensitive to bright sunlight. This problem can be treated with a simple operation that replaces the damaged lens with a plastic one.

The build up of glucose and sugars in the small blood vessels that supply the retina makes them weak. Small blisters can form and occasionally burst, resulting in tiny haemorrhages. This is called diabetic retinopathy. In recent years, laser treatment has been developed to repair the damage it causes.

Feet

Diabetics must pay special attention to the care of their feet and look for changes in the shape of their feet. They should always wear shoes that fit properly. Periods of high blood glucose can cause damage to the nerves in the body (see page 25), particularly the feet, making them less sensitive to pain and temperature. This means that people with diabetes may not notice accidental injuries or infection. For this reason they should wash and check their feet every day. If any ulceration is noticed they should seek medical advice immediately.

Skin

There are some potentially serious skin problems related to diabetes. If diabetics notice any changes in their skin they should see a health professional immediately. In most cases, these skin problems can be managed with early diagnosis and treatment.

▲ *People with diabetes are advised to make daily inspections of their feet. They should see a chiropodist annually who will check their ability to feel pressure on the soles of their feet and toes.*

Fungal infections can occur in the hands, feet, groin and vaginal areas. Fungi feed on high glucose levels and so diabetics are more susceptible to infections. The skin is a favourite site for fungi to flourish. Infections can cause severe itching and discomfort, as well as looking unsightly. Fungal infections can be controlled with anti-fungal creams and treatments.

Diabetic dermopathy usually occurs in skin that has been injured or traumatised. It appears as round, brown or purple, slightly-indented patches of skin, most frequently found on the shins. It tends to occur in people who have had diabetes for at least 20 years. It can be treated with low doses of zinc prescribed by a doctor.

Necrobiosis lipoidica is a disease of the legs that can be very disfiguring. The skin over the lower shin bones becomes thin, showing broken blood cells and inflamed redness. It only affects one in 300 people with diabetes, but women are three times more likely than men to be affected. There is no known treatment, but good blood glucose control will prevent it from occurring.

Other health issues

If people with diabetes take good care of themselves and keep their blood glucose within normal levels, it is unlikely that their condition will lead to other complications. However, problems can occur in the heart, kidneys and nerve system from prolonged periods of high blood glucose levels.

Heart

Heart disease is quite common in people with diabetes. The arteries around the heart are at risk of narrowing if blood glucose levels are not kept under control. Diabetics are advised to eat a low fat diet and not to smoke because of the increased risk of heart disease. Eating healthily and taking regular exercise will help to keep the heart healthy.

▼ Having high blood glucose levels over a long period of time can cause problems with the heart, kidneys and nervous system.

Brain connected to central nervous system

Arteries and blood vessels supply oxygen around the body

Heart pumps blood around the body

Narrowing of the arteries can cause problems with blood supply to the heart.

Pulmonary artery

Renal artery carries blood with waste products to the kidney

Renal vein carries cleaned blood

Kidneys filter waste products from the blood

Ureter carries waste products (urine) to the bladder

Kidneys

The job of the kidneys is to filter waste products from the blood into the urine and to keep protein inside the body. A build up of glucose in the blood vessels can damage the kidney's filtering system and cause protein to leak into the urine. This means that waste products may build up in the blood causing further damage. If left untreated, the problem will escalate and may lead to dialysis treatment being required. Regular urine tests can detect the problem at an early stage and, with treatment, the kidneys can recover completely.

Nerves

Nerve fibres are made of very long, thin cells. After many years of diabetes, these cells can be damaged by a build up of glucose in the blood, which deprives them of oxygen. If affected, a person becomes less sensitive to pain and may experience numbness or tingling. The feet are the most vulnerable, but tenderness caused by nerve damage can also be felt in the hands and shoulders. Impaired sensitivity to pain means a person with diabetes may seek medical attention for a wound later than they would otherwise. This gives more time for infection to arise.

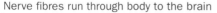
Nerve fibres run through body to the brain

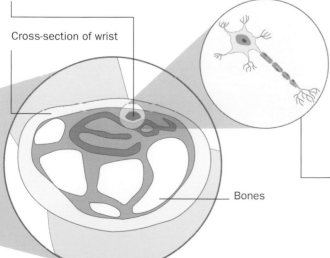
Cross-section of wrist

Bones

Nerve cells send sensory signals to the brain and can become damaged by high blood glucose levels

MANAGING WHEN ILL

Diabetes Australia give this advice to people with diabetes who become ill: 'Everyday illness or infections will nearly always cause a rise in blood glucose levels whether you have Type 1 or Type 2 diabetes. Therefore, at the earliest sign of any form of illness, such as a cold or virus, it is important for you to take action.'

People with diabetes who are feeling unwell should:

• NOT stop taking their insulin or diabetes medication.

• drink plenty of unsweetened fluids, aiming for about five pints a day.

• try to replace the usual amount of carbohydrate by sipping sugary drinks or sucking glucose tablets if they cannot eat solid food and are worried about having a hypo.

• test their blood glucose level regularly to ensure it is not too high. If blood glucose levels are over 15 millimoles per litre, or urine tests are positive, they may need to increase their dose of tablets or insulin.

• seek medical advice if blood glucose levels are continuously high, they are vomiting and unable to keep anything down or they are unsure what to do.

Healthy eating and drinking

A healthy diet is important for everyone. As children and adolescents are still growing, their diet is especially important. All children should have regular check-ups to make sure they are the right weight for their height. This is especially important for children with diabetes.

Planning ahead

People with diabetes need to plan what they are going to do each day and think about when and what they eat. They need to remember to carry extra insulin when necessary, for example if they are going to a party and may be eating lots of food. They also need to eat regular snacks to ensure there is enough glucose in their blood for their insulin to work on.

Carbohydrates

Carbohydrates are our main source of energy. We should eat enough carbohydrates to give us energy throughout the day, especially if we are going to do sport. It is also important to do enough exercise to use up all the energy from the food we eat. If you take in more energy than you use, the excess carbohydrate will be stored as fat and can make you overweight. This can cause other health problems.

▶ *Carbohydrates are an important part of a healthy diet. They are also an important source of glucose.*

Fatty and sugary food

Everyone should avoid eating too many fatty and sugary foods. Sugary snacks put a lot of sugar into your bloodstream quickly. For diabetics this can be a problem as it may cause their blood glucose level to go too high. Eating fatty and sugary foods occasionally should not be a problem as long as people with diabetes adapt their insulin doses accordingly.

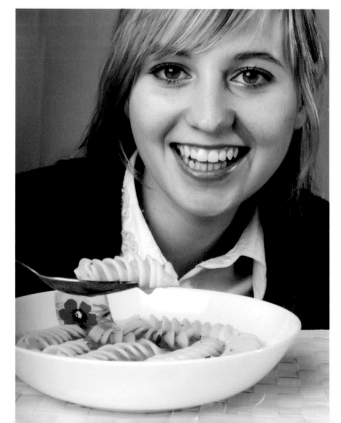

There are snacks that are made especially for diabetic people, such as diabetic chocolate, which is made with sweeteners rather than sugar. However, these foods often contain a lot of fat and may cause diarrhoea. Artificial sweeteners are a good substitute for sugar as they do not affect glucose levels. They can be used to sweeten food and drinks. Sugary drinks such as glucose drinks, cola, lemonade and orange juice are digested quickly and this is why they are recommended when blood glucose levels are low.

Vegetarians

If an effort is made to achieve a balanced diet, diabetics can be vegetarian. They should make allowances for the high sugar content of certain fruits, such as berries, and take care to avoid vitamin and mineral deficiencies. This may mean eating more of certain foods or taking a vitamin supplement. Diabetics are advised to talk to their doctor or a dietician before following a vegetarian diet.

Fasting or missing a meal

Some religions have times of fasting, such as Yom Kippur for Jews and Ramadan for Muslims. During such times, people with diabetes must monitor their blood glucose levels frequently and adjust insulin levels accordingly. Insulin should not be cut out altogether. Diabetics are advised to talk to their doctor or a dietician before fasting.

▶ *It is important to eat plenty of fruit and vegetables every day. Some studies have suggested that eating fruit and vegetables can help reduce the risk of Type 2 diabetes.*

CASE NOTES

EVETTE'S STORY

Evette Stacey is 37 and lives in the UK. She was diagnosed with Type 1 diabetes when she was 29. She says: 'You don't need to follow a specific diet, but you do need to have a good, healthy diet, much the same as someone who doesn't have diabetes. I eat plenty of fruit and veg and keep my intake of fats, sugars and salts in check. I suppose the only thing I have to do differently is to understand how the food I eat affects my blood glucose.'

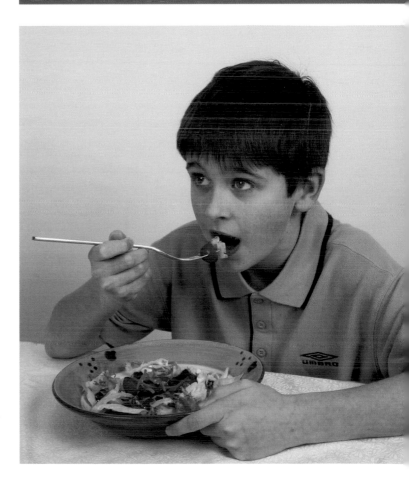

Physical activity

Diabetics are able to do any sport if they take the necessary precautions. Exercise will especially help Type 2 diabetics if they are overweight. For a diabetic who takes short-acting insulin, regular exercise can improve insulin sensitivity even after they have finished exercising.

Preparing to do sport

Diabetics must prepare themselves for exercise by eating properly and checking their glucose levels. If they know they will be doing some form of exercise within a few hours of eating, they may need to eat a little extra or decrease their insulin intake. It is advisable to avoid strenuous activity for two hours after taking insulin.

Exercise lowers blood glucose levels by increasing the amount of glucose absorbed into muscle cells. This is because your muscles need energy during exercise. It is a good idea for diabetics to take a blood glucose reading before they start exercising,

▼ *Good diabetes management means that diabetics are able to do sport to whatever level they are comfortable.*

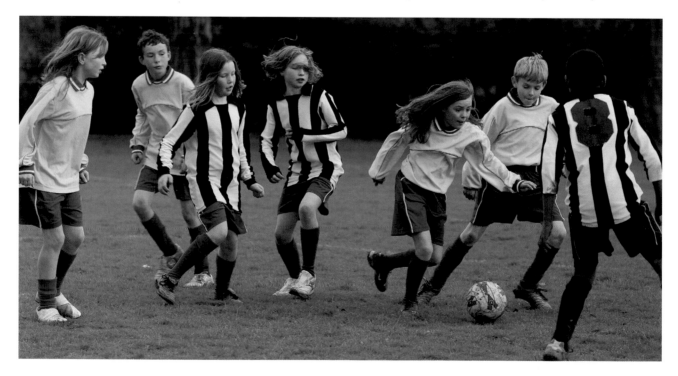

and to top up with glucose drinks or snacks as necessary. After exercise, the muscles will have increased insulin sensitivity for up to 48 hours. Insulin doses may need to be lowered for up to 36 hours after exercise to prevent a hypo.

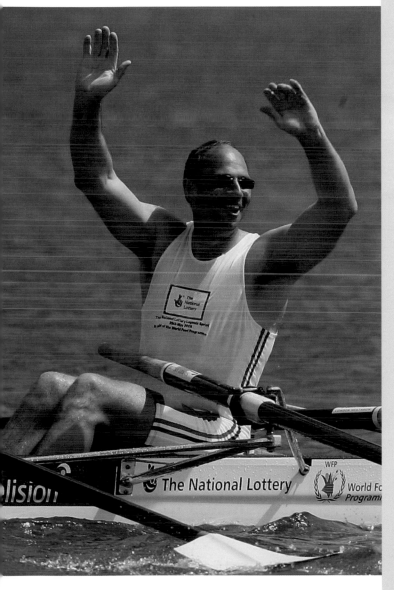

▲ *Olympic rowing champion, Steve Redgrave, has Type 2 diabetes. He has proved that it is possible for someone with diabetes to lead a healthy life with few limitations.*

CASE NOTES

STEVE'S STORY

Steve Redgrave is five times British Olympic rowing champion and was the first athlete ever to win five gold medals in endurance events in successive Olympics. He was diagnosed with diabetes when he was 35. He put his body through rigorous training, yet still kept good control over his diabetes and reached a peak physical fitness.

'The first telltale sign was a terrible thirst after training, which I could only quench with pint after pint of blackcurrant juice. When we went on training camps overseas, we were given dipsticks to test our urine for dehydration. I had some lying around the house so I tested myself and was positive. Next morning, further tests by a doctor revealed my blood sugar levels were sky high. Within hours of seeing a specialist at Wycombe General Hospital diabetic clinic I was injecting insulin to regulate my blood sugar.

When I was first diagnosed in 1997, I was completely devastated and, initially, I believed that I would no longer be able to continue training for the Olympics in 2000. How wrong was I? I soon realised that, with special guidance and support, I would be able to continue training and reach the goals I had set myself. Now, I use a fast-acting insulin every time I eat, which works out at six jabs in the abdomen a day.'

Living with diabetes

Diabetics have to learn how to incorporate their condition into their everyday life. Diabetes does not stop people doing what they have always done or want to do. By taking precautions, they are taking control of their diabetes, and not letting it control them.

Having a daily routine

Being diagnosed with diabetes may be overwhelming at first. Sometimes people feel burdened by the number of tests and insulin doses or tablets they must take. Diabetics may find their condition easier to control if they stick to a routine. They should test their blood glucose before and after a change in routine, for example, if they miss a meal or take part in a strenuous exercise class. They should always carry extra snacks in case there is an unplanned change in their daily routine. Diabetics should also ensure the people they are with know where their snacks are and how to treat a hypo.

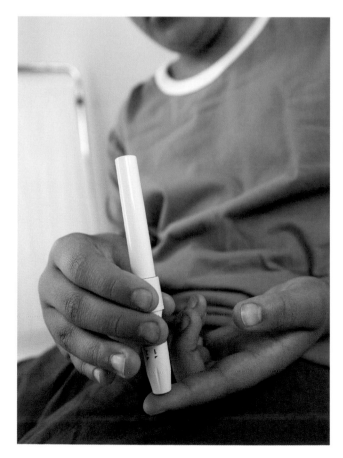

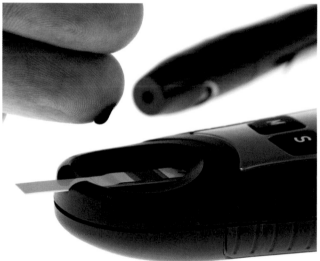

◀▲ People with diabetes are taught how to monitor their blood sugar level. This includes using a blood glucose meter, like the one above, to test a drop of their blood. From this they will be able to tell if they need more insulin.

Understanding emotions

Fluctuations in blood glucose can cause mood swings and heightened emotions. People with diabetes are three times more likely to suffer with depression. The loss of control over their own body can also affect a diabetic's self-esteem and cause anxiety, leading to stress. Regaining control over the situation will give them back their confidence. There are many online forums or local support groups where a person with diabetes can share their experiences and talk about their emotions. Sharing the burden can reduce stress and help a person take control.

FAMOUS PEOPLE WITH DIABETES:

Sir Andrew Lloyd Webber, musical composer

Billie Jean King, tennis player

Ernest Hemingway, 20th century novelist

H G Wells, writer

Halle Berry, actress

James Cagney, producer, director and actor

Johnny Cash, legendary country singer

Meat Loaf, singer

Menachem Begin, Israeli prime minister

Thomas Edison, inventor

MEDIC ALERT

There are special medical alert chains, like the one below, that people with medical conditions, like diabetes, can wear. This has a symbol that is recognised all over the world and any medical staff will know that the person has a medical condition. This may help when treating them.

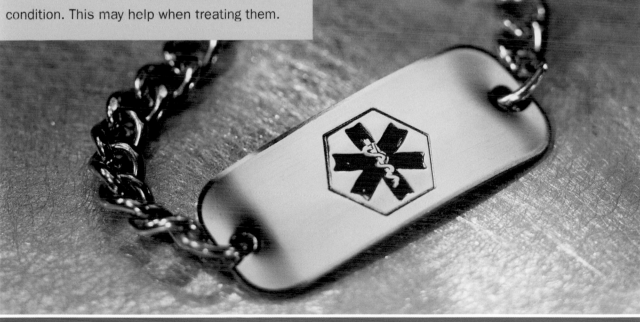

Diabetes and families

Diabetes is hereditary, meaning it runs in families. There is more chance of children having diabetes if their parents have it, or even an uncle or aunt. People with diabetes may learn to cope with their condition better if a close relative also has the condition and can give them advice. Knowing someone who also manages the condition can be very comforting.

Family life

When a close family member has been diagnosed with diabetes, life will inevitably change. Diabetes affects the whole family and impacts on family life.

For young people and adolescents, the normal sorts of conflict that accompany growing up may become magnified, with diabetes becoming a source of strife in the family. Teenagers may resent feeling so dependent on insulin and fight for more independence by not following their regime. This may be normal behaviour for teenagers but, when centred on diabetes, this can be very dangerous. Refusing to take their prescribed insulin injections or tablets can increase the risk of other health problems.

▼ *Teenage mood swings can affect the whole family. If you feel angry or upset, then talking with family members can help.*

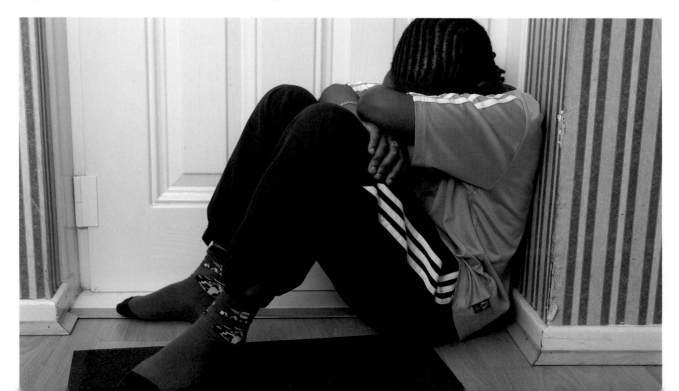

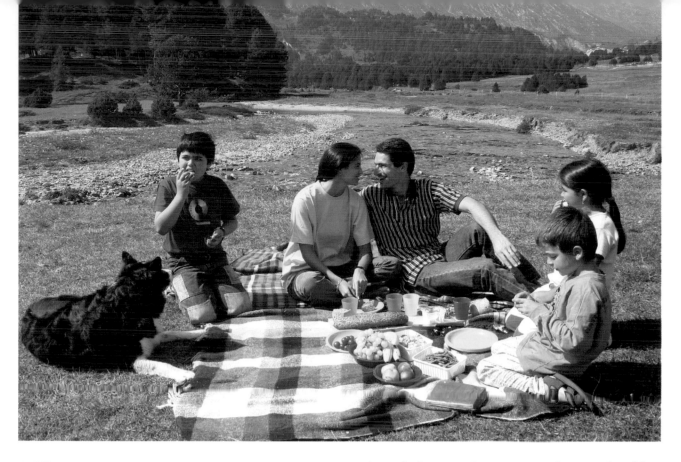

▲ *When planning ahead for a family holiday, people with diabetes need to consider such things as where they are going, how long they are going for, whether they will be more active than usual, and if they will be eating out.*

Parents

Parents of children with diabetes may find they are faced with the dilemma of how to be supportive without being too over-protective. They must ensure that they do not unnecessarily give diabetes as the reason why their child may not do things. For example, when refusing a snack before dinner they should say it would ruin the child's appetite, whether they have diabetes or not.

Siblings

If you have a brother or sister with diabetes it may be frustrating to see them getting more attention than you, and you might feel left out. However, if you have diabetes you might get fed up with all the attention and feel like people are always checking on you. You might feel jealous of a brother or sister without diabetes as they can eat whatever they like, and do not have to keep checking their blood glucose and taking injections or tablets. If you do feel angry or upset with siblings or parents you should always talk to them about it, as they may be feeling upset too. Talking together can help you all understand your feelings and plan changes to improve the situation.

Holidays

Diabetics can travel all over the world. As long as they plan ahead they can have an enjoyable and safe trip.

Lee's mum, Cecilia (see page 13), explained, '*If we go somewhere very hot then I always make sure there is a mini-fridge in the room so we can keep Lee's insulin at the right temperature. I also make sure we have plenty of glucose tablets in case we can't get them in the country we are in and ensure we have enough insulin with us, as it wouldn't be very easy to get some if Lee ran out or lost his.*'

Diabetes at school

Diabetes should not be a problem at school. Diabetics, or their parents, should make sure that teachers and other staff understand what diabetes is and what to do in an emergency.

Support at school

Younger children with diabetes will need support when they start school and it is a good idea for their parents to have a meeting with staff beforehand. Parents should also provide spare insulin and syringes, spare snacks and a glucagon kit to be kept in a safe place at the school.

As diabetics get older, they learn to manage their diabetes effectively at school themselves. Staff and friends should still be made aware of their medical needs and should know what to do if a child with diabetes feels unwell, or develops hypoglycaemia.

Children with diabetes need to be allowed to go to the bathroom frequently and have access to water when required, especially when their glucose level is high. Diabetics should carry a snack or glucose tablets with them during school hours. Teachers need to be aware that following a hypo it can take several hours to fully recover. It is important that a pupil having a hypo is not left alone, or allowed to wander off or run away. Schools may ask a specialist diabetes nurse to give a talk about diabetes so that everyone is aware what the condition is and how it is managed.

▼ *Diabetes does not stop young people from following and achieving their dreams.*

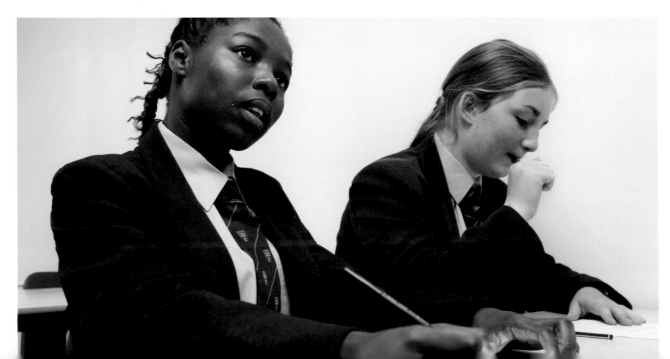

Lunchtime

Diabetics should ensure they eat properly while at school. Regular meal times should be established, with lunch at the same time every day. When eating lunch from the school cafeteria, a person with diabetes should check that there is something on the school menu that they can eat. If there is nothing suitable on the menu they should allow enough time to arrange an alternative.

Physical Education

When timetabling PE lessons, teachers should consider when a diabetic child takes their insulin injection or tablets and what time they usually eat breakfast or lunch to reduce the risk of a hypo. The child will also need to be allowed to have an extra snack before or after PE.

Exams

Stress before an exam may cause blood glucose levels to be higher. If difficulties are experienced during an exam, a diabetic should measure their blood glucose level. If the results are not normal, they could be used as evidence if the exam needs to be taken again. Diabetics should also be allowed to eat something during an exam if they need to.

School trips

Going on a school day trip should not cause any problems, as long as the routine is much the same as at school. The child with diabetes should have their insulin injection or tablets as usual. They should also carry their glucose snacks and take their glucagon kit, just in case.

CASE NOTES

KATIE'S STORY

Katie is fourteen years old. She found out she had Type 1 diabetes when she was nine. She checks her blood glucose level three or four times a day.

'At school, I hate being late for lunch because I'm checking my blood sugar and insulin. I always worry about checking my blood sugar and taking the right amount of insulin and having enough snacks and then I worry what other kids will think when they see me doing all these things.

I don't want anyone to treat me differently. Okay, I admit, I might occasionally use the 'diabetes card' to get out of something I don't want to do, but very, very rarely.

My life is like an onion: I have all these layers of things that complicate the day, like going to parties, and school, getting my homework finished, and dealing with my parents. Then there is diabetes, which adds an extra layer to everything. I know I have the worries of every other teenager but then I have the added worry of diabetes. Looking at my diabetes as just another layer helps me to put my life into perspective.'

With overnight stays, parents need to be confident that children are able to do injections on their own, or that there is a member of staff who is willing to take responsibility for helping with injections and blood glucose testing.

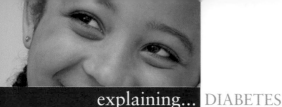
Growing up with diabetes

At present there is no cure for diabetes. It is therefore a lifelong condition.

As people with diabetes grow up, they will find there are new challenges to face.

Puberty

Diabetes can be affected by the way young peoples' bodies change during adolescence, and they will need a lot more insulin. During puberty, insulin treatment needs to be looked at and modified regularly. This means that check-ups are especially important during this time.

People with diabetes also need to make sure they are the right weight for their height. If they do not get enough insulin, they will lose weight and may not grow as they should. If they get too much insulin they will gain weight.

Leaving home

Leaving home can give young people a greater sense of independence. People with diabetes may feel a greater sense of self-esteem and confidence when they are able to manage on their own. Diabetics should take into consideration that once they move into a place of their own they will have to take sole responsibility for their diabetes.

Alcohol

When people grow up, they may want to drink alcohol in social situations. Alcohol contains carbohydrates which initially raise blood glucose levels. However, alcohol also prevents the liver from releasing glucose, and so may increase the risk of a hypo by lowering blood glucose, especially if the stomach is empty. There is no reason why

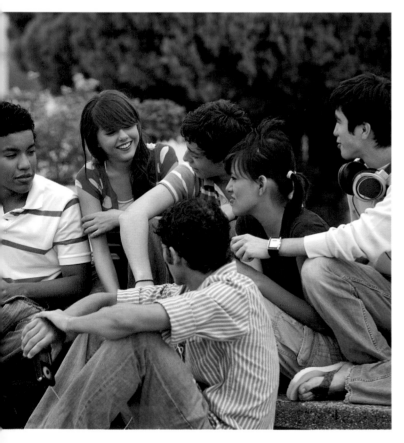

◄ *Young people who want more independence must learn to manage their diabetes themselves. Well controlled diabetes should not interfere with a young person's social life.*

young adults should not drink alcohol if they have diabetes as long as they do not exceed the recommended amounts.

Getting a job

Having diabetes does not mean that you cannot get or keep a job. In many countries there are laws which protect people with disabilities from discrimination in the workplace. Almost all types of employment are open to people with diabetes. Usually diabetics can adjust their insulin doses to fit with working hours and shift patterns.

However, a person with diabetes should think seriously about their condition when choosing a career. Some jobs, such as an airline pilot or professional driver, may not be suitable because, if they became hypoglycaemic, they would be putting other people's lives at risk. It is advisable to seek career advice before leaving school.

ADVICE ON DIABETES

Robert Skinner is 58 and was diagnosed with Type 2 diabetes three years ago. His advice is: 'Only you can manage your diabetes – you don't have to go without things you love all the time, but eat pretty healthily, do some enjoyable exercise, enjoy the odd drink, get regular check-ups – and love life and yourself – and you'll live to a ripe old age! I intend to!'

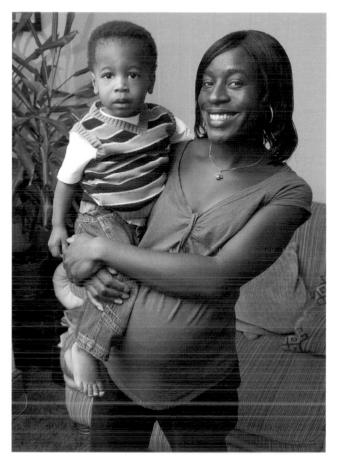

▲ *Women with diabetes are able to have healthy children.*

Having children

Diabetes does not prevent people from having children. Pregnancy can be more difficult for those with diabetes and they should take extra care to control their blood glucose before and during pregnancy. They should discuss their pregnancy with their doctor who will be able to give advice about whether they need to change their medication or take extra supplements. With the right care and management of blood glucose levels, women with diabetes are able to give birth to perfectly healthy babies. If a parent is diabetic there is a greater chance that their child will also have diabetes.

The future for diabetes

New treatments for the effects of diabetes have improved greatly in recent years. Successful kidney and pancreas transplants are bringing hope to people with organ failure, while medical technology and new ways to administer insulin are being tried and tested all over the world.

Pancreatic surgery

Pancreas transplants have been performed for many years, often at the same time as kidney transplants, as the risk of the body rejecting the new organ is lower. If a pancreas transplant is successful there is no need for any more insulin injections, but other medicines must be taken to prevent rejection.

Artificial pancreas

Research is being conducted into combining insulin pumps (that are currently used by people with Type 1 diabetes) and continuous glucose monitors that will work together to monitor and regulate insulin doses automatically. This works as an artificial pancreas and is proving to be very effective.

'The artificial pancreas combines two pieces of technology – an insulin pump and a continuous glucose sensor, which provides real time data about trends in glucose levels and alarms the patient to intervene if levels are heading too high or too low.' Juvenile Diabetes Research Foundation UK (www.jdrf.org.uk)

Blood glucose meters

Glucose meters have made home monitoring much easier. The next generation of monitors that

AN INSULIN PILL

Scientists from the National Tsing Hua University in Taiwan have announced they are developing an insulin pill to replace daily injections.

'Further testing of this [pill] is needed to determine its suitability as an insulin delivery system – a goal that is some years away. However, our research is taking us a significant step forward towards this important goal and offering hope to people who are living with diabetes,' said Dr Colin Thompson, Research Fellow at the university's School of Pharmacy.

Libby Dowling, Care Advisor at Diabetes UK, said: 'Oral insulin could make a big difference to the lives of people with diabetes. Children, elderly people and those with a phobia of needles would benefit particularly if and when insulin capsules become a safe and effective treatment for the condition.'

are being researched use infrared light to measure glucose levels. This means that levels can be measured without taking blood samples.

CATHY'S STORY

Cathy is 49 and was diagnosed with Type 1 diabetes when she was five years old. She talks here about having an islets of Langerhans transplant.

'I was offered the chance to have an islets of Langerhans transplant. It is still a relatively new procedure, but the result for me has been superb. After the first transplant my insulin intake went down and I had fewer hypos. Then after the second transplant, seven months later, my insulin intake was further lowered and I had no hypos at all! The result is that for the first time since the age of five I know what it is like to feel well on a long-term basis. It is glorious. I have been given back my health, which is the most precious thing we have.'

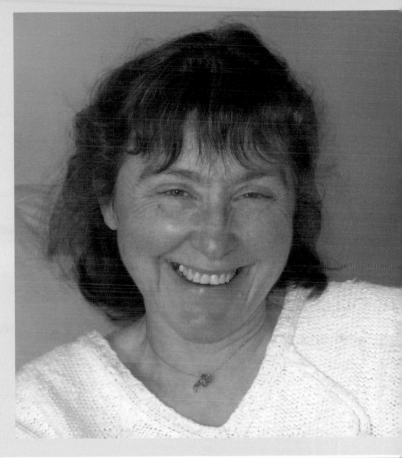

Insulin delivery

Experiments in taking insulin through an inhaler have been trialled on adults and children over the age of twelve. The insulin is absorbed quickly through the lining of the lungs and lasts like short-acting regular insulin. However, some episodes of severe hypoglycaemia have been recorded. It is not recommended for people who also have asthma and has not yet been approved for all children and adolescents.

Scientists are also looking at taking insulin as a nasal spray so that insulin can be absorbed through the lining of the nose. However, problems arise if a person has hay fever or gets a cold. There are also concerns about how the insulin will affect the lining of the nose with long-term use. For this reason it is not yet a clinical reality.

Research has also been conducted into islet cell transplants (see *Cathy's Story* above). The islets of Langerhans can be extracted from a donor and injected into the liver of a person with diabetes. The person will then be able to produce their own insulin. So far however, only 12 per cent of recipients have been able to manage without insulin injections for more than a week. All islets research has been conducted on adults with diabetes.

Glossary

adolescence the time when a young person develops into an adult

auto-pen a device that people can use to inject insulin easily, it looks like a pen and contains a thin needle which is inserted under the skin to inject insulin

blood glucose level the concentration of glucose in the blood, measured as the number of millimoles of glucose per litre of blood

blood test a test in which a small sample of blood is taken; this can be done with a syringe, or by pricking the finger and squeezing out a drop of blood

carbohydrates the main food group that gives us energy; this includes bread products, cereals, potatoes, rice and pasta

cataracts when the lens of the eye becomes cloudy and makes a person's vision blurry

chiropodist someone who specialises in feet

contagious when an illness or disease can be caught from someone else who has it

cystitis inflammation of the urinary bladder, caused by an infection, that makes it painful to pass urine

dehydrated a lack of water in the body which causes a feeling of weakness

diabetic a person who has got diabetes

diagnosis identification of a disease or condition after careful examination of the body and symptoms

dialysis treatment people with kidney problems have dialysis treatment, which filters their blood as their kidneys normally would

diet the food a person regularly eats

dietician someone who advises people about what to eat

fungal infection an infection caused by fungus

fungus a group of organisms that feed on organic matter

genetically engineered changing an organism's genetic material to enhance or subdue certain characteristics

glucagon a hormone produced by the pancreas that stimulates an increase in blood glucose level

glucose a type of sugar that is found in certain foods and is turned into energy inside the body

glycaemic index (GI) a figure representing the ability of a food to raise blood glucose levels; low GI means that a food does not raise the body's blood sugar level too much

haemorrhage when a blood vessel breaks and allows blood to escape

hereditary passed from parent to child

hormone a chemical made by one part of your body that causes a change or reaction in another part of your body

hypoglycaemia (hypo) the reaction a diabetic has when their blood glucose is too low (below 4 millimoles per litre)

injection when a fine needle is used to insert medicine into the body

insulin the hormone produced by the pancreas that helps the body to covert glucose into energy

islets of Langerhans small cells in the pancreas that produce insulin

laboratory a room containing special equipment to be used in scientific experiments

millimoles per litre measurement used to calculate blood glucose levels

monitoring regular tests and observations done to ensure that blood glucose levels stay normal (between 4-6 millimoles per litre)

opaque cloudy, not able to be seen through

palpitations a noticeably rapid or strong heartbeat

pancreas a gland that produces hormones that help the body to digest food

physiologist a scientist who studies how parts of living organisms work

puberty the time when a body changes from a child's to an adult's

recovery position a position used in first aid to prevent choking in an unconscious person

retina a layer of cells at the back of the eye that are sensitive to light

retinopathy a disorder that affects the retina in the eye, and is caused by many years of high blood glucose levels

seizure a sudden fit or attack when a person loses control of their body

symptoms changes in the body that indicate that a disease or other condition is present

thrush an infection of the mouth and throat, or genitalia, by a yeast-like fungus

ulceration when skin becomes infected by an ulcer, an open sore on a surface of the body which fails to heal

urinary tract the channel through which urine leaves the body

urine test a sample of urine taken for testing

virus a tiny organism that multiplies in a body's cells, often causing disease

zinc a metal that is found in many foods that is essential for proper nutrition

Further information

Books

Coping with Diabetes,
Pat Kelly, *Rosen Publishing Group, 2000*

Diabetes (Health Issues),
Jo Whelan, *Wayland, 2003*

Diabetes (Diseases and Disorders Series),
Barbara Sheen, *Lucent Books, 2003*

Diabetes,
Margaret O Hyde and Elizabeth H Forsyth,
Franklin Watts, 2003

Diabetes (Twenty-First Century Medical Library),
Marlene Targ Brill,
Twenty-First Century Books, 2007

Diabetes (Contemporary Issues Companion) ed.
Louise I Gerdes, *Greenhaven Press, 2003*

Diabetes (Feeling Sick),
Jillian Powell, *Cherrytree Books, 2008*

Diabetes (Frequently Asked Questions),
Judith Levin, *Rosen Publishing Group, 2007*

Diabetes (Need to Know),
Jenny Bryan, *Heinemann Library, 2005*

Diabetes (Perspectives on Diseases and Disorders),
eds. Tom Metcalf and Gena Metcalf,
Greenhaven Press, 2007

Diabetes Snacks, Treats, and Easy Eats for Kids,
Barbara Grunes, *Surrey Books, 2006*

**Diabetes: The Ultimate Teen Guide
(It Happened To Me),**
Katherine J Moran, *Scarecrow Press, 2004*

Diabetes (What Does It Mean To Have),
Louise Spilsbury, *Heinemann Library, 2002*

How I Feel: A Book About Diabetes,
Michael Olson, *Lantern Books, 2005*

Juvenile Diabetes (Health Alert),
Johannah Haney, *Benchmark Books, 2005*

Juvenile Diabetes,
Jason Glaser, *First Facts Books, 2006*

**Living with Diabetes
(Living Well: Chronic Conditions),**
Shirley Wimbish Gray, *Child's World, 2002*

Living with Diabetes (Teen's Guides),
Katrina Parker, *Checkmark Books, 2008*

Living with Diabetes,
Jenny Bryan, *Wayland, 2005*

My Friend has Diabetes,
Anna Levene, *Chrysalis Books, 2003*

Why Me? Why Did I Have To Get Diabetes?,
Robert Messinger, *Little Mai Press, 2004*

Websites

www.bbc.co.uk/health/conditions/diabetes

BBC webpage that gives information on Diabetes and has personal stories from people with the condition. It also has a list of useful contacts for people who need more information.

www.childrenwithdiabetes.com

US site with lots of useful information and links to similar sites all over the world. Hosts its own forum and chat rooms where young people can share stories and make friends.

www.diabetes.co.uk

UK site that has a lot of information and a special section for young people.

www.diabetes.org

Website of the American Diabetes Association that gives lots of information for parents, teachers and kids about diabetes.

www.diabetescamps.org

US Diabetic Education and Camping Association website. It mainly contains information about camping holidays for children with diabetes based in the USA but, there is an international camp directory featuring similar camps from all over the world.

www.kidsdiabetes.co.uk

A website set up by a girl with diabetes who gives lots of information about living with diabetes.

kids.jdrf.org

Kids section of the Juvenile Diabetes Research Foundation (JDRF) website designed for kids with diabetes and their friends and family. Lots of information about diabetes and news and information about current research that JDRF are doing.

Note to parents and teachers: Every effort has been made by the Publishers to ensure that these websites are suitable for children, that they are of the highest educational value, and that they contain no inappropriate or offensive material. However, because of the nature of the Internet, it is impossible to guarantee that the contents of these sites will not be altered. We strongly advise that Internet access is supervised by a responsible adult.

Index

These are the list of contents for each title
in Explaining:

Asthma

What is asthma? • History of asthma • Increase
in asthma • Who has asthma? • Healthy lungs
• How asthma affects the lungs • What triggers
asthma? • Asthma and allergies • Diagnosing
asthma • Preventing an attack • Relieving an attack
• What to do during an attack • Growing up with
asthma • Living with asthma • Asthma and
exercise • Future

Autism

What is autism? • Autism: a brief history • The rise
of autism • The autistic spectrum • The signs of
autism • Autism and inheritance • The triggers of
autism • Autism and the body • Autism and mental
health • Can autism be treated? • Living with
autism • Autism and families • Autism and school
• Asperger syndrome • Autism and adulthood •
The future for autism

Blindness

What is blindness? • Causes and effects
• Visual impairment • Colour blindness and night
blindness • Eye tests • Treatments and cures
• Coping with blindness • Optical aids • Guide
dogs and canes • Home life • On the move
• Blindness and families • Blindness at school
• Blindness as an adult • Blindness, sport and
leisure • The future for blindness

Cerebral Palsy

What is cerebral palsy? • The causes of cerebral
palsy • Diagnosis • Types of cerebral palsy • Other
effects of cerebral palsy • Managing cerebral palsy
• Other support • Technological support •
Communication • How it feels • Everyday life
• Being at school • Cerebral palsy and the family
• Into adulthood • Raising awareness • The future

Cystic Fibrosis

What is cystic fibrosis? • A brief history • What
causes cystic fibrosis? • Screening and diagnosis
• The effects of cystic fibrosis • How is cystic
fibrosis managed? • Infections and illness • A
special diet • Clearing the airways • Physical
exercise • Cystic fibrosis and families • Cystic
fibrosis at school • Living with cystic fibrosis •
Living longer • New treatments • Gene therapy

Deafness

What is deafness? • Ears and sounds • Types of
deafness • Causes of deafness • Signs of deafness
• Diagnosis • Treating deafness • Lip reading
• Sign language • Deafness and education
• Schools for the deaf • Deafness and adulthood
• Technology • Deafness and the family
• Fighting discrimination • Latest research

Diabetes

What is diabetes? • Type 1 diabetes • Type 2
diabetes • Symptoms and diagnosis • Medication
• Hypoglycaemia • Eyes, skin and feet
• Other health issues • Healthy eating and drinking
• Physical activity • Living with diabetes
• Diabetes and families • Diabetes at school
• Growing up with diabetes • The future for diabetics

Down's syndrome

What is Down's syndrome? • Changing
attitudes • Who has Down's Syndrome?
• What are chromosomes? • The extra
chromosome • Individual differences
• Health problems • Testing for Down's Syndrome
• Diagnosing at birth • Babies • Toddlers
• At school • Friendships and fun
• Effects on the family • Living independently
• Down's syndrome community

Epilepsy

What is epilepsy? • Causes and effects • Who has
epilepsy? • Partial seizures • Generalised seizures
• Triggers • Diagnosis • How you can help
• Controlling epilepsy • Taking medicines
• Living with epilepsy • Epilepsy and families
• Epilepsy at school • Sport and leisure
• Growing up with epilepsy • The future for epilepsy

Food allergy

What are food allergies? • Food allergies: a brief
history • Food aversion, intolerance or allergy?
• What is an allergic reaction? • Food allergies:
common culprits • Anaphylaxis • Testing for food
allergies • Avoiding allergic reactions • Treating
allergic reactions • Food allergies on the rise • Food
allergies and families • Food allergies and age •
Living with food allergies • 21st century problems
• The future for food allergies